Curve Appeal

How to Lose Weight and Feel Great in Your 30s, 40s, 50s, and Beyond

By Lorraine Peters

www.TheCurvyCoachLorraine.com

Photo of Lorraine Peters on the front cover was taken by Rachael Peters

ISBN-13:978-1511958158

Health and legal disclaimer

This book is not intended as a substitute for the medical advice of physicians. The reader should regularly consult a physician in matters relating to his/her health and particularly with respect to any symptoms that may require diagnosis or medical attention.

I. Natural Health

II. Fitness & Dieting

III. Diets & Weight Loss

Your Free Gift

As a way of thanking you for purchasing *Curve Appeal*, we'd like to offer you a supplementary article not found in this book. This article deals with how to select "worthy goals". Since the content of this book covers the topic of behaviour change we thought you'd also appreciate this article which will further enhance the information provided in the book. You can download your guide by going to

www.thecurvycoachlorraine.com/goals

Acknowledgement.

I want thank my Husband Randy for his generous nature as I continue to explore who I am. Everything that I have accomplished in my life, including this book, is largely due to the unwavering support and unselfish ways of this wonderful man.

Foreword by Kim Hunter

Author Lorraine Peters pens an unabashedly raw account of how one chubby young girl, blossomed into a healthy, fit and happy champion of clean eating and exercise. She takes the reader through a very simple and straightforward method of losing and maintaining an ideal weight based on her own personal struggles. She finds the silver bullet starting with "strength of commitment." In a nutshell, she shows how a winning attitude and the ability to get back on track after momentary lapses is the key to winning in the long-run. In her many years as a Fitness Trainer and Wellness Coach, she uses her former clients' successes and failures as a guide to demonstrate that success comes to those who commit to long term and consistent behavior and healthy eating changes. An advocate of fitness and regular exercise she also demonstrates the connection between a healthy mind and a healthy body! Curve Appeal is an easy read, and both a compelling story of one woman's life-long efforts to maintain a healthy weight, as well as a how-to guide for the reader to follow. It is NOT your mother's diet book – but one you'll want to gift to your girlfriends. It has given me a renewed attitude and desire to change my own lifestyle.

Kim Hunter is a Saint John businesswomen, friend, and former client who admits to drinking too much wine!

Do you want sustainable, long term weight loss?

The pain of yo yo dieting, weight loss and repeated weight gain, is caused by not understanding the reasons why you overeat and not committing to a lifestyle of healthy food. Your days of fad diets and weight gain will be solved if you follow the advice of this book. We'll cover your personal wellness vision, barriers to success, tips for changing behaviours and setting healthy goals so that you will learn how to lose weight and keep it off forever. My experience is in the areas of simple "can do" behaviours, which taught me that it is possible to achieve a balanced lifestyle and weight without extreme measures that don't last. *Curve Appeal* will teach you practical and sustainable ways to eat that fit into your life and for these reasons you will never ever diet again.

Table of Contents

CHAPTER ONE: Through thick and thin

My first memory of not fully expressing my personality because of my weight was at the age of eight; my friends and I were in our bathing suits, standing outside my parents' car waiting to go swimming and they were all wearing bikinis. I was not.

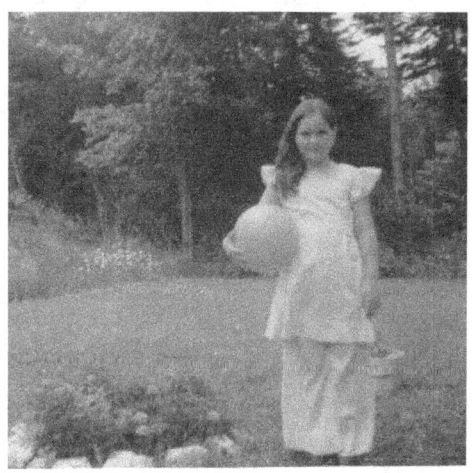

I love fashion and clothing, so it's no surprise to me now that my first memory of being overweight had to do with clothing. I was consumed with thoughts of how they could wear their bikinis so effortlessly, and how they could be so oblivious to the reality that not everyone could wear them. I would have swum the English channel to look good in a bikini. I looked at those girls like they were superheroes or, at the very least, really special, and probably smarter because they could wear a two-piece. All these thoughts were tumbling in my head while I waited to go swimming. Wow, I'm tired just writing about it.

As I grew up I was very good at convincing everyone that I was comfortable with being bigger than my peers, but in reality I was jealous of them all. I secretly mourned the things I knew I would not do, and wear, because of my weight. I would have given anything to look like them, and to experience what seemed to be the ease of movement and self expression that accompanied being slim and trim. Healthy eating was not even discussed in my youth as a means to a slim, bikini-worthy body. It would be many years before I would discover the power of food.

You see, despite the many millions of dollars that we spend each year on diets that promise to be the best, and that will make you thin and keep you that way, most of them focus on the food itself. Most books and methods focus on the author's viewpoint on eating certain foods at certain times while this book will focus more on the mindset of the weight loss process, meaning that if we can gain perspectives about our health and our weight situations, we can begin to think differently in order to change how we act.

Back then, my mindset was very different than it is today; I don't remember how old I was when I first heard the term big-boned, but I liked the sound of it, and was thankful to have one saving grace. I was pretty and I knew how to dress to look my best so now to have something to blame my size on, like my bone structure, was fabulous. Since the reference to my bone size came from my family, I took it as the God's truth. In high school I even had a tough girl reputation because of my size 14 frame. I guess it had its advantages after all! Not.

I'll never forget the image of my friend Carole (we met when I was 16) walking down the hill toward my house on a hot summer day. It had been about two weeks since I had seen her, and I couldn't believe my eyes; she must have lost 20 pounds and was so thin. To me, she looked so good and it didn't matter to me how she did it, I just wanted to know how. I was shouting on the inside, tell me how! In the early '80s there were not a lot of diet aids on the market, and definitely none to be found in the small Canadian town that bordered the USA where I grew up. Carole told me she had taken diet pills; wanting the same results, I set off on a cross-border trip to purchase the same little miracle in a box that worked so well for her. My foray into pill-assisted weight loss didn't work because I soon realized that you also had to go on a very low calorie diet. Not prepared to starve myself, I quit. I guess subconsciously I always knew that was the wrong approach.

Still 16 and still looking for the easy fix, I moved onto the world of diet shakes. There was one very popular new brand so, once again, I headed across the border to purchase it. Those didn't work either because I found it too much work to follow the specific diet that came with it. With each failed attempt to lose weight I became more and more convinced that my family was right, that I was big-boned. And those big bones were the reason I was destined to be a size 14 forever.

At the age of three I knew I wanted to be a model. I know what you are thinking, "Could this girl torture herself any more?" and "She's overweight but she chooses a path where everyone is rail thin!" I was pretty enough, but instead of being a size 4, I was a size 14. In the early '80s there was an emerging new trend which the fashion world pegged as the full figure model. The industry had finally recognized the need to make clothes for women who represented the size 12-and-up segment of the population. At age 19 I went to a modelling and finishing school outside Toronto; it was a wonderful experience that taught me how to walk, apply makeup professionally, go on calls for jobs, photo shoots and all that other model stuff. I absolutely loved it. I finished the course and went on calls for modelling jobs but ended up moving home to be close to my family. Soon after returning home I developed and taught a self-improvement course for young girls in my hometown, and life went on.

The most vivid memory relating to my weight happened when a complete stranger saw right past my pretty face and called me fat. I was horrified. The word kept ringing in my head, over and over and over. I pretended that I was unaffected by it though, because I was out with friends, and because at the time I was still hiding behind the big-boned definition of my body. I had made it to my early 20s and it was the first time I had ever been called fat. Someone I didn't even know said what I had known all my life but I had never heard it verbalized by anyone before.

I was never the same after that night. Being called fat did something to me. I knew in that moment that some people viewed me as not just a bigger girl who was pretty, but rather as a girl who was overweight. Two years after the name-calling incident, I was sitting around the table with three friends who were also somewhat overweight and unhappy with their bodies. We were talking about weight loss, and became determined to do it together. I can remember like it was yesterday how serious I was about leading this group of girls to join a local program as soon as possible; with everyone in agreement we joined Weight Watchers™.

The Weight Watchers program completely changed my life. I was so diligent in tracking my food, just like the leader had taught me. I never missed a meeting, and I made every single recipe that was on the program. I did not deviate one bit. It took me one year to lose 35 lbs, going from a size 14 to a trim size 9/10. I clocked in at a healthy and lean 150 lbs on a 5'6" frame. This was all accomplished by diet alone. I had not yet been bitten by the exercise bug but when I discovered exercise my life would never be the same. The exhilaration I got from exercise was like being born again. I was a different person.

Losing 35 lbs literally transformed me into a new person. The old me was still intact, but the person I had always wanted to be was finally on the outside. I was wearing my thin-side on the outside and it felt amazing; no longer was my thin-side stuck inside where only I could imagine her potential. Two years after losing the weight, I became a certified fitness instructor. Exercise had become a major part of my weight loss success, and I loved how it made me look and feel. Now I was ready to teach others. Becoming a fitness instructor changed my life and it would shape the future for me in ways that I could not imagine at the time.

The first group fitness class I taught was Aquacize, or water aerobics. Now, as you know, in order to teach Aquacize you must first slip into a bathing suit. I will never forget how it felt to be standing on the pool deck in my Speedo leading a fitness class! The music blasting, I was jogging in front of 20 people, and I was perfectly comfortable. To this day I love getting up in front of a group of people to teach any kind of fitness class, and it's a great example of how I fully express myself because I am now comfortable and confident with my body. I would never have had this wonderful experience if I still weighed 185lbs.

Being fit and slim allows my authentic self to shine through, and it is the fundamental reason why I know that when people say "I'm fat and happy" it's a lie. It may be what they need to tell themselves until the time arrives and they're ready to change, but it is still a lie. When you live a life where you do not feel comfortable to express exactly who you are, there is no way you can ever be happy.

I had not modeled at all since I had left it behind in my late teens, but I was offered a chance to model wedding gowns and jumped at the opportunity. Fit, toned and wearing a size 9 wedding dress, I felt like a supermodel and to this day I cherish those photographs. I went on to enjoy modelling for a couple of years; one distinct highlight was the request to model in the annual world buyers fur show in Montreal. The week away from my nine year old son was the longest we'd been apart and upon my return he greeted me at the door with 'Mom' written across his forehead in permanent marker. After this I took a long leave from modelling but in my late 40s was asked to step back into modelling bridal wear and as I'm writing this chapter, I am preparing to travel to a nearby city for another fashion show.

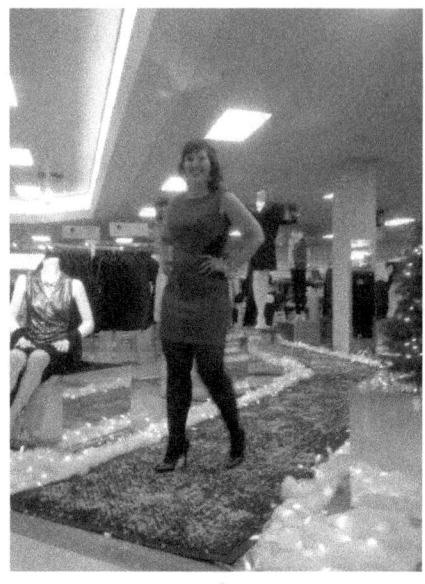

I have often thought about who I would have become if I had lost weight as a young girl, what doors might have been opened, what opportunities and experiences might have been mine. But there is no sense crying over spilled milk and with each new adventure as a slim and fit person, my world was changing and unfolding in ways I always envisioned it would. The life I was now experiencing and the new positive way I saw myself was accomplished because I had become fit and slim!

It was becoming clear that fitness was going to play a major part in my life, both personally and professionally. Those early years as a fitness instructor were so very special to me because although I had a full-time career in sales I had this incredibly fulfilling side job as a fitness leader. In the early '90s fitness classes like step aerobics were wildly popular; I can recall teaching classes with 60 or more participants. The facility that I taught in (and still do on occasion) was the Canada Games Aquatic Center, and back then it was a badge of honour to be one of their fitness instructors. We were all certified through what was at that time the N.B Council for Fitness and Active Living, a provincial body governing and insuring fitness instructors in New Brunswick. Between 1994 and 2005 I continued to take courses in fitness and to nurture the dream of pursuing it as a full time career but in the interim I enjoyed it for what it was: an awesome hobby that helped keep me fit and healthy.

As an overweight child and teen I secretly liked the idea of lifting weights, and had somehow managed to take possession of a weight bench, leg curl and barbell, all tucked safely in the basement of my parents' home. I would use the set from time to time but didn't have the knowledge or resources to learn or keep me motivated so I never made any real progress with it. I was also interested in arm wrestling and was quite good at it too. One of my father's friends was a fitness buff of sorts and followed the arm wrestling circuit in the US. I remember him telling me that he'd met - and wrestled - a female arm wrestling champ and was amazed at how strong I was compared to her. Even though I was not athletic and I never did pursue arm wrestling, I had a desire to compete in a bodybuilding competition. Growing up in rural Charlotte County in the '70s and '80s I felt I may as well be striving to be the first woman on the moon; it was simply a far-fetched and likely unattainable dream. It would be more than 20 years before my dream was actualized.

In 1992, the same year that I began my weight loss journey, I met my now-husband Randy. Randy was and still is the most supportive person in my life, always believing in me even when I didn't believe in myself. As women, it is so important for us to have men like this in our lives, men who admire and uplift us because life is difficult enough without surrounding yourself with people who don't have your best interests at heart. Eight years later, in July '99, we were married and shortly after that I set my sights on having more children. My son Ryan was four years old when Randy and I met; Randy is the only father Ryan has ever known and the bond between them is very strong. A year later I conceived and quickly settled into a pregnancy mindset, remaining very active during the entire pregnancy but not monitoring or restricting my food in any way. My weight soared, and post-delivery I was 220 lbs. I remember standing on the scale, looking down at the number and saying to myself 'here we go again girl'. It had been nine years since I lost the extra weight and I had kept it off but now I was looking at a number on the scale that was 35lb heavier than the weight I started at back in 1992.

Even though it seemed like a daunting and overwhelming task I immediately started watching what I ate, omitted sugar and reduced my intake to about 1300 calories per day which is within the standard caloric range for most women who are moderately active and want to lose weight. Within a couple of weeks of having my baby I was back teaching fitness classes at the local Y but was so heavy that I strained all the tendons and ligaments in my feet and ended up with painful plantar fasciitis. It took about a year to completely heal and be pain-free but with every 5 lbs that I would lose I could feel the stress on my joints and feet being lifted; being overweight is so hard on your body, in every way. My slow-and-steady-wins-the-race attitude was paying off once again and after about a year my weight was down to 175lb and I was feeling good! It was about this time that Randy suggested that we have another baby, since we'd had Rachael when I was 37 and now, a year later, it felt like time was running out.
I became pregnant immediately and this time I vowed to keep my weight in check and within the healthy limit for pregnancy weight gain. My desire

and intentional approach to not gain unnecessary weight during my third pregnancy paid off, and I stayed below the 200 lb mark. This success was hugely gratifying and it taught me that when it comes to successful weight loss you must reach a point where you want the weight loss more than you want the instant gratification of the food. Having iron-clad motivation is vital to reaching your goal. After giving birth to Raye-Anne Meadow, I acknowledged she was my last baby and set my sights on getting my body back.

I needed a BHAG! This acronym was coined by one of my favourite educators of all time, Bob Tchannen-Moran. It stands for 'Big Hairy Audacious Goal' and boy did I have one of those. In fact I'd had this goal since I was a teenager. I was going to compete in a bodybuilding competition! Less than 1% of people will ever step onto a bodybuilding stage. I don't know exactly where that statistic came from but the purpose of it being said to me was to drive home the reality of just how difficult it is to get onto that stage in peak form, wearing a bikini so small it comes delivered in a plastic sandwich bag, both pieces!

I vividly recall standing in the checkout at Walmart, eight months pregnant, lumbering and tired, pointing out the cover of an Oxygen magazine to my mother (for those not familiar with Oxygen and Robert Kennedy Publishing, it is, in my opinion, the best resource for fitness and clean eating on the market). I said to my mother "I'm going to do that" and she looked but had no idea what I was talking about so she responded "Do what?" I explained that I was going to compete in a bodybuilding competition and she simply remarked "I see". I'm certain that it was a shocking claim from someone who was weeks away from childbirth, hovering just under 200 lbs and clocking in at 39 years of age. My mother is wonderful and supportive in every way but this was hard for even her to envision. I don't hold it against her!

Once I had that beautiful baby girl in my arms I set my sights on once again getting the weight off. I now had two girls under the age of two, as well as a teenage boy. My weight loss was slow but constant and I was healthy and energetic. By late 2005 I was ready to start training and focusing on a competition and I put my trust in a young man named Adam Walker. Adam was a firefighter by day, with a successful after-hours supplement business on the outskirts of the city. When I first met Adam and told him I wanted to compete in a bodybuilding competition he was very supportive and encouraging, even optimistic. My start weight was 173 lbs and once I began 'eating clean' (a fitness industry term) the weight just fell off. I had decided that I would step on stage for a show in my own city on June 30, 2007; this gave me nine months to train hard and diet down to the low weight and low body fat that is required to be competition-ready.

The process of bodybuilding broke down so many of the limiting beliefs that I'd held about myself. The least I had ever weighed was 148lb and I can still remember the day the scale hit 145lb; it was not the weight that meant so much to me, rather it was what the weight represented. I now knew with certainty that if I simply ate clean consistently, day after day, I could achieve my lowest healthy weight. There was nothing that could have made me believe it except for living the reality day in and day out, and then seeing the results for myself. I knew from that moment on that the false and limiting beliefs from childhood I'd clung to about myself and my body were simply not true. I was not big boned, and I was not destined to be a size 14, size 12 or even a size 10.

Bodybuilding has taught me that the single most important aspect of losing weight is consistency: one hundred percent of people who eat clean food, eat it every day, and allow a small treat once a week or on occasion will reach their weight loss goal, one hundred percent of the time. This philosophy has become the primary tenet by which I coach my weight loss clients. They must accept the reality that if they want to achieve a slim and fit body they must be consistent - not perfect, just consistent.

The reason I am telling you this is because too often I see clients who eat clean for four or five days only to eat badly all weekend and maybe consume some alcohol as well. If they continue the on/off cycle they soon become frustrated because they do not see the weight loss results so discouragement sets in and they quit. That's the cycle of inconsistency. In your mind you're thinking you have been good and only cheated a little bit but in reality it was just enough extra calories to prevent any weight loss from happening.

Bodybuilding also meant that surrounding myself with like-minded people can be very motivating; when you are feeling down and can't imagine carrying on, it is great to have a mentor, friend or coach to get you back on track. It's unrealistic to want to lose weight but then surround yourself with people or environments that do not reflect your goals. The best way to achieve a slim fit physique is to associate with slim and fit people. You cannot achieve a lean fit body if you live a sedentary junk food-filled life. The two cannot coexist.

My hope for you as you read my book is that you find yourself nodding your head in understanding because as difficult as it was to write down how I was feeling when I was an overweight kid, I want readers to feel like they can relate. I want you to know that it doesn't matter, at all, what your past was like; anyone, absolutely anyone, can change their body and attain a healthy body weight if they really want it.

Understand that you became overweight because of the way you think, the resulting behaviours, and the day to day reality of eating too much food and probably the wrong kind of food. If you are to reverse this, you must accept new and different behaviours, actions and thoughts to totally transform your body. You cannot change your weight situation using the same techniques that got you fat. You must change your way of living if you are serious about losing weight.

CHAPTER TWO : Not everyone will grow with you

You are going to experience the cold shoulder from some people as you begin your healthy lifestyle changes and choices. Even people who love you may not like this new you, with your sudden penchant for healthy food and regular visits to the gym. As much as it's an adjustment for you it is also an adjustment for your close circle of family and friends; to some extent the person with whom they shared countless unhealthy meals and bad habits is forever gone, resulting in resentment and a sense of loss by those closest to you.

As you begin to explore this new world you will meet new people who support your goals and with whom you share a common interest. Family and friends who do not share your desire to have a slim fit physique and healthy body are going to feel left out and left behind, they will feel they have nothing in common with you as you focus intently, especially in the beginning, on changing your bad habits to good. You may even find that you begin to distance yourself somewhat from these individuals - and that's okay. Not only is it okay, it is actually necessary if you are to be successful with long term weight loss and maintenance. You must commit to doing what you need to do to make this work for you. If you plan to successfully lose weight and keep it off, you are going to have to change your behaviours, attitudes and old thought patterns about food, exercise and living in a health-promoting way. It's not just for a few meals or a few hours each day; it is a mindset of health and wellness that's in place all day, every day.

There is very little difference between how you must eat to lose weight and how you must eat to maintain your weight so you need to embrace the notion of living healthy every single day. This shift in how you live will undoubtedly result in losing some friends along the way. It may be a mutual and subtle parting of the ways, or in some instances, relationships fall away more abruptly. I have had many clients feel guilty about this. They feel that they are becoming health snobs, traitors almost, and turning their backs on old friends now that they are healthy but what's really happening is more like a growth spurt. You are out-growing the activities of that group of people, and you realise you want something different. It doesn't mean that the way they are living is bad, it just means that you choose to move in a different direction.

One of my leisure activities is driving my Harley Davidson. I have many biker friends whose company I really enjoy, and some of them live the biker lifestyle. They like to party often, and eating healthy and getting adequate sleep is not a way of life for them. It would be so easy to fall into this pattern if I allowed myself to be around it too often but I don't; I make a conscious effort to honour what is most important to me which is my health and wellness. My plan is to live well and healthily to at least 100, so partying to excess and not taking care of my body will not help me reach my vision. It is the same for you. You don't have to throw away long time friendships or family but at the end of the day you have to honour your vision for your health and fitness.

I had a client who was a nurse at the local hospital. She was bright and I'm sure the other nurses that she worked with were intelligent people too. When my client was well into her weight loss journey, her station put on a birthday celebration for a co-worker complete with Chinese food and a beautiful big fluffy cake. My client offered to pick up the cake, bring it to the party and participate but said she was not going to indulge in any of the birthday food. Her co-workers gave her such a difficult time about not eating the lovely food that a colleague had specially made, and why wouldn't she have a small piece of cake... how bad could it be? By the time the party ended my client was in tears and couldn't understand why it bothered her so much. It bothered her because she was being bullied! The other nurses were threatened by her resolution to eat clean - while they sat around and ate their body weight in cake and Chinese food - because it forced them to take a good look at themselves and their weight, and that was uncomfortable. So they took it out on her.

This or something like it will happen to you, I guarantee it. Someone will gently coerce you into eating some cake or having a piece of pizza or having just a bit of wine. It's so important that you prepare for these sabotaging scenarios and have a script ready. You should remain polite but firm when you tell people that although you do have something special to eat from time to time, this event is not the time that you choose to go off your clean eating plan. I strongly recommend that you reach out to meet new people who have an interest in fitness and weight loss too. There is so much motivation and strength when you are surrounded by like-minded people

Please don't think I'm suggesting that you trade in all your family and friends for new ones now that you are losing weight and regaining your health! I'm simply giving you a heads-up that it is perfectly okay if some relationships don't grow with you.

This is an exciting time for you, enjoy it and embrace new possibilities for growth!

CHAPTER THREE : The mindset of weight loss: six surefire tips for success

Despite the many millions of dollars that we spend each year on diets that promise to be the best, and that will make you thin and keep you that way, most of them focus on the food itself. Most books and methods focus on the author's viewpoint on eating certain foods at certain times while this book will focus more on the mindset of the weight loss process, meaning that if we can gain perspectives about our health and our weight situations, we can begin to think differently in order to change how we act.

Ideally, every person on earth would know what they have to do to be relatively fit and at a healthy body weight but unfortunately that's not the case. I always say that if the only client I had was the one who really did not know what they should be doing I would be out of business because there is so much more to weight loss and healthy living than knowing what to do. That's where I come in.

We are in a new millennium and the rules have changed. Why? Because the circumstances in which we live and by which we eat have changed. In the chapter '5 Pillars of Weight Loss' we discuss how we can't apply the same techniques to weight loss when our life situation or body chemistry changes, how we have to approach our goals of weight loss and health differently if we are to be successful. Adopting and consistently following this list of six actions and behaviours will ensure your long term weight loss success. Remember that your thoughts create feelings and your behaviour follows. Change the way you think and feel and you can change the choices you make.

1. Surrender to the Process

We cause our suffering when we feel like we are being deprived of something that we really enjoy, like eating and drinking. It all becomes easier - much easier - if we surrender to the process of losing weight. Take a moment and let those words swim around in your brain. What do I mean by that, surrender to the process? I was struck by this bolt of enlightenment when training for my very first bodybuilding show, with the realization that once I surrendered to the fact of how I had to eat and exercise to make this dream come true, it suddenly made it much easier. It was easier to keep reminders of my goals in front of me on the fridge and on my vision board as a reminder of exactly why I was doing this. I was not prepared to wake up every single day of life wishing I could have a chocolate bar or a sandwich - it was a waste of energy and time.

So I embraced the life and actions of a bodybuilder, competed and won. As I carried this experience forward to my clients, I began to see that the clients who fully accept the lifestyle they have to live if they want to achieve a healthy body weight, do so much better than those who want to lose weight but are always flirting with weekend drinks and having dates with ice cream. On weigh day they come prepared for battle - with themselves. It is this self-sabotaging behaviour that makes us feel bad about ourselves; it leads to harmful negative self-talk and further reinforces our false belief that we simply can't do it. We can't do it because we have neither surrendered to, nor fully accepted, the way we have to live and eat to actually achieve the goal.

Self-efficacy is the belief in one's own ability to complete tasks and reach goals. And, interestingly, once you adopt a consistently healthy way of living and you see results on an ongoing basis you begin to build self-efficacy, and confidence in your abilities to achieve set goals. On the flip side? Every single time you do not honour what you say you want for yourself, you erode your belief in your ability to achieve it. Now take a minute to read that last bit again - every single time you do not honour what you say you want for yourself, you erode your belief in your ability to achieve it.

2. Mindfulness and Presence

What would you say if I told you that I had just invented a fantastic pill that would 100% guarantee that you would lose weight faster and keep it off longer than if you did not take it? Heck yeah, give me a truck load! Well, as much as people fight the act of journaling, tracking or writing down their food intake, it has been proven to be the single best action to ensure not only quicker weight loss but also that the pounds stay off. Why is journaling food intake so powerful yet resisted by so many? I have heard many different reasons over the years, ranging from I can't remember, to I only write down when I've been good, to I just hate doing it. The best one was 'it makes me feel like I'm obsessing over food too much'... oh really? You don't want to know the rest of that conversation!

We need to journal because as much as we think we can remember everything we put into our mouths we simply cannot. Not only what we eat but also how much, since portion control is a significant element in the plan to regain health and fitness. If you are reading this and muttering under your breath that you're one of those people that CAN remember everything you eat... no, you can't. If you could, you wouldn't be in this situation to start with. If you are not committed to tracking every single item that you put into your mouth you may as well put this book down now, because success will elude your every effort without the required mindfulness.

Journaling is a conscious acknowledgment of what you just ate, and how much. It registers in your brain and forces you to remember it. If you write down absolutely everything it becomes a running tally that you can reference to be reminded of how you ate yesterday or last week, and it gradually reveals its positive purpose: when you have a really good week or month of weight loss and you get to wondering why it went so well you can look back and see how you ate. It enables you to easily repeat that positive behaviour. Twenty five years ago when I lost 30lb I did it with the Weight Watchers program; they taught me the habit of food tracking and I've done it every day of my life since. I track my food, my water, my exercise, as well as my mood and mindset (happy, sad, tired etc.)

It doesn't matter how you journal. I personally enjoy a nice hard cover journal and a pen but you can use electronic means as well, from iPhone to Android, Notepad or computer. There are plenty of great free online journaling resources now, with a particularly popular choice being myfitnesspal.com.

Final words on mindfulness and presence: if you bite it, write it; if you nibble it, scribble it. Be in the moment and never ever eat on the run - sit down, even if it's for two minutes. Mindfulness also means being in the moment when you are eating. I know sometimes life is hectic with very little time for sitting around doing nothing but you must take time to eat in a mindful and conscious way. When you do this it gives your brain and stomach a chance to realize that you have eaten. If you just inhale your food while you are working, watching TV, driving or performing other tasks you won't enjoy it or taste it, and your brain won't recognize that you've eaten so you are likely to eat more, eat more often and consume far too many calories. Sit down, eat your food, enjoy every bite then continue on with your day.

3. Accountability

In nearly 20 years in the business of fitness and weight loss I have not figured out why women think they have to do this on their own. On countless occasions I've seen women struggling and they will say "I know what to do. I should be able to do this on my own" and then six months later they are still saying the same thing. Why, why, why? I don't understand why, if you are struggling with something for a long time, it is so hard to reach out for help. If you were drowning, would it be a sign of weakness to reach for the life jacket? If you were facing bankruptcy, would there be shame or weakness in seeing an expert in the area of bankruptcy? If you were getting married, would there be shame in seeing a wedding planner? Is there weakness in consulting a retirement planner to help you get the most money possible for your retirement years? No. No. No. No. So why this attitude of solitary confinement when it comes to your weight?

I mentioned previously that if the only client I had was the one that truly did not know what to do to lose weight then I'd have no clients... and maybe that's the issue. Intellectually, women understand what they must do to lose weight but doing it and sticking to it is the problem. Perhaps it's because the notion of having a personal trainer or nutritionist is seen as frivolous spending of hard-earned money. From time to time I've heard married women say that their husbands don't understand why they have to see a personal trainer or nutritionist to lose weight. "Just stop eating," they say. I'm here to tell you that it's more complicated than that.

Accountability is a crucial part of the weight loss journey that should never end. You need some sort of support to get you through the bad days, you need a resource that is stimulating you and motivating you to carry on. You need accountability; that little voice that says you are going to have to check in with this person or that group so you better stay on track. Again, some people view this as being overly-consumed or obsessed with weight loss but if you have struggled with your weight for many years and tried many different approaches, you definitely need ongoing accountability and support. This is why the Weight Watchers program is so darn successful; it is the attendance at meetings and the learning and group support that keeps people coming back.

There are many ways to ensure accountability: perhaps a buddy (just make sure it's someone who is not going to let you off the hook), a group environment (local weight loss group) or even a group of girlfriends who want to lose weight together. Online tools are popular these days and there are "group" options on those programs as well so you can be part of an e-group. It should not be your significant other because they may find it difficult to convey honesty in a way that you will accept and find useful. It is also easier for us to manipulate our partner or get mad at them when they are attempting to hold us to our goals. Just like journaling, I am not so concerned about how you do it as long as you do it. Find some avenue by which you are held accountable to the goals you have set for yourself.

4. Consistency, the Golden Rule
In my practice I say this word so often that one of these days someone is going to throw something at me! Here's a newsflash for you: any diet will work. There, I said it. I'm not talking about how healthy they are because in my opinion some diets are harmful, but for the sake of this conversation I am stating that any diet will work. You will lose weight if you follow absolutely any of the diet books on the shelf today because the difference between success

and failure in losing weight is consistency. You do not have to be radical or extreme in your approach, and you don't need to live on cabbage soup and exercise five hours a day to lose weight. If you are an average active woman, you need to consistently consume 1300 calories each day from healthy vegetables, fruit, fats and protein. It is that simple. If you are a man who needs to lose weight I recommend no less than 2000 calories each day.

Consistency becomes key to weight loss when we are in our mid-30s and older because our bodies no longer respond to radical and extreme attempts to lose weight. Gone are the days when you could step on the scale, not like what you see, then binge your way back down to your happy spot in three days. That's unhealthy anyway but more importantly your body does not tolerate such radical action as you get older, and responds best to the slow-and-steady approach instead. Strive to be 90% on plan at all times and you will be successful in your weight loss endeavour.

Here's a great analogy to drive home the power of consistency in weight loss. I want you to picture a large locomotive. We all know how much energy and time it takes for that train to get up to speed on the track, and we also know that once the train gets up to speed nothing can stop it - in fact, it takes a lot of energy and time for that train to come to a stop once it's going full tilt. Now picture that same train having to stop and start, stop and start, stop and start. It would never get any momentum, would it? Exactly. And that's what I want you to acknowledge, that consistency leads to momentum and momentum leads to consistent weight loss. When you continuously stop and start you never gain momentum and then you get frustrated because you don't see results so you become demotivated and quit. Sound familiar? And to think a simple thing like consistency is the culprit.

5. Clean environment

To this point, everything we've discussed has not really involved anyone except you but that's all about to change. When it comes to the mindset of weight loss, a big part of it is having a clean environment. You may have watched this take place on some of the popular weight loss shows where the nutrition coach visits the subject's home and systematically goes through all the cupboards and refrigerator to throw away the bad food. There are a lot of worthwhile reasons for this exercise so let's get started. Think about a time when you are particularly vulnerable to overeating or emotional eating; it may be 9pm and you've struggled through a long hard day and now find yourself with a craving for unhealthy munchies and let's face it, your first pick will not be a salad or a chicken breast. Right? You rifle through every pantry shelf until your eyes land on something that makes your heart flutter... you practically inhale it, barely chewing, stuffing until finally that awful Oh what did I do feeling sets in and the regret starts bubbling up.

I can see you nodding your head in intimate understanding of the scenario I just described. How different would this scene have been if there were no bad snack foods in the house at all? What if you had to get up, get dressed and go out to the store and buy the junk food? What is the likelihood that you would have done that? And even if you did, you would have been far more likely to give it some thought before picking out food, taking it to the checkout and paying for it, driving back home and THEN after all that, eating it. This last scenario provides you many opportunities to think about it and reflect on what your goals are for losing weight and then ultimately fighting the temptation to not do it.

The problem with having junk foods or trigger foods in your house is that you don't stop and think about your goals and all the reasons why you shouldn't eat the junk, and instead just go for it and regret it horribly after the fact. Many people resist purging their homes of junk food because of their spouses or their children. Why are you keeping junk food in your home for the sake of others? I'm assuming that eventually you want to improve the health and fitness of everyone in your home so eliminating junk food from your house should be a given, even if no one has a weight problem. In my house if we want a treat we have to physically go out for it. That's just a rule I have. If my kids want something at the store then they walk to the store to get it. Nine times out of ten they don't bother. Isn't that great?!

If you are resisting cleaning out the junk food because of the resistance from your spouse then I would recommend this approach. In a non-emotional manner sit your partner down and have a little heart-to-heart. Help the person to see that you are absolutely determined to lose weight, and that one of the biggest challenges will be the temptation in the kitchen cupboards. Most can appreciate what a very real threat the junk food poses for you and will be more sensitive and supportive. Together, brainstorm solutions that will make both of you happy.
In an ideal situation I don't want any trigger foods in your house whatsoever but if you have to come to a compromise with others in your house I would recommend that any such food items be in a room and in a container that you don't even know about, and in a location that is a real inconvenience for you to access. Much like driving to the store, it would provide opportunity for you to reconsider your impulses and evaluate the triggers. In my experience with clients over the years, the willingness to create a completely clean home environment is directly proportional to their commitment to their weight loss goals. Much like journaling, a clean environment is a

clear signal of your desire to reach your weight loss goal.

6. Motivators and Values

To be successful with long term behaviour change you must give thought to your motivators for weight loss, the values you have in your life, and how losing the weight supports that which you value in your life. The more heartfelt and meaningful the motivators, the more likely you will be compelled to stick with your plan to lose weight. You will less likely be swallowed by the buffet table if you are reminded of why you are doing this. Being mindful at all times of why you are changing bad habits for good will ensure that you stay on the right track.

CHAPTER FOUR : Managing Expectations

By now, everyone knows that there is no magic diet pill that will make you skinny. Without effort on your part, it can't happen. Thanks to a tremendous amount of science and research in the field of nutrition and exercise, we know more about the way the body works during exercise and how it utilizes nutrition than ever before, making this the best time in history to achieve the body you desire. You just need to know the facts so you can move forward, armed with the knowledge required to make the changes you want in your body.

It's important to acknowledge the difference between what you want and what you are willing to do to get it; it is important to be realistic about these two (sometimes different) goals. We frequently invite unnecessary stress into our lives by wanting and desiring something that we have no intention of earnestly pursuing to the point of actually achieving. That's wasted energy, so stop it!

In my practice as a personal trainer and wellness coach I always screen potential clients by offering a complimentary consultation. Sometimes people say they want to weigh 125 lbs like they did back in high school but they hate to exercise and they won't eat vegetables. That's where I remind them I'm a trainer, not Merlin the magician! Seriously though, you have to consider whether your goals are based on the reality of your lifestyle, and if you will do what you need to in order to achieve them. Is it that you would like to be slim but you really aren't willing to do what it takes to get slim? Or is it that you would do anything to lose weight but you just need a good program to follow? The latter is preferable.

When I was an amateur bodybuilder I lived very clean; I did not drink alcohol, I did not eat sugar, I carried a large cooler of my food everywhere I went and yes, I enjoyed single digit body fat but I'm not willing to do that anymore. I'd love to look that way - who wouldn't - but I'm no longer willing to do what it takes to look like that. Nowadays, my goal is to stay fit and wear a single digit clothing size but I also want to enjoy my social life, and that includes an occasional glass of wine and my favourite food.

I encourage you to give thought to what you want for yourself and your body. What is your ultimate goal or vision? Describe your ideal self. How do you look and feel, what do you value in your life that is supported by making healthy lifestyle changes? What are the advantages of making healthy changes? What are the disadvantages of those same healthy changes, because there are always disadvantages - you may have to miss social engagements because you don't feel you can be around the food and alcohol, or you may need to get a good night's sleep to get up early and hit the gym. Add up the pros and cons for yourself; ideally, the advantages column will be stacked higher with the benefits of becoming more fit and healthy.

CHAPTER FIVE: Alcohol and Weight Loss

Where to start! For many of us alcohol is something that we relate to leisure time, as a symbol of dedicated time to ourselves or relaxing with family and friends. The peace and quiet we've been waiting for all week, when a drink is a marker of relaxation and doing absolutely nothing, and that moment you are able to put your work day aside and head to your favourite watering hole or pub for that magical first sip of beer or wine. Aah it's great isn't it? I get it, really I do.

Whatever the scenario, it is unrealistic for most people to commit to zero alcohol consumption but at the same time it is important to understand that there are several key factors affecting weight loss that are related to alcohol. If you choose to maximize your weight loss then you may have to omit alcohol from your life entirely for a while; when your goal weight is reached, you could add it back in modest amounts. The primary approach of those who are trying to lose weight is to consider only the caloric value of their alcoholic drinks, and use only this factor in assessing the potential damage to their diet plan. Below I share a range of additional factors for consideration that will make you knowledgeable, and put you in the position of making an informed decision using all the facts.

Calories

Most regular beer contains about 150 calories while light beer has about 80. Most hard liquor is approximately 150 calories per ounce, with the same applying to the average glass of wine. If you are adhering to 1300 cal/day you can see how only a few drinks would put you over your daily limit, creating an even bigger problem for those who enjoy the fancy cocktails made with juice, fruit and syrups. You could easily be consuming 300+ calories in one cocktail.

Decreased inhibitions

Drinking impairs judgment and disables defenses, at least somewhat. If you are drinking and there is food around you are more likely to graze or pick at food without being aware of the mindless nibbling. If you are unaware of the food you are consuming then you are not tracking it and you are going to be over your daily calorie intake for weight loss. Quick tip: always eat your healthy food before you go to the party and make a conscious plan to move yourself far away from the food tables.

Metabolism

After consuming 4 oz of alcohol your metabolism slows down, meaning all of your bodily functions that utilize calories for energy also slow down.

Essentially it means that if you were burning say, one hundred calories doing nothing before you consumed the alcohol, you suddenly burn far fewer calories after consuming 4oz of booze. Drinking alcohol prevents the body from losing weight in the way it usually would if you weren't drinking.

Exercise
Some may not feel very energetic the morning after the night before thanks to staying up past their usual bedtime, or as a result of consuming too much alcohol. In my experience people are generally far less active than they normally would be, and instead of getting up and out or going for their workout or even a walk they may opt instead for lying around watching a movie and napping. You don't have to be a math wizard to figure out that you are not going to lose weight without expending energy through exercise.

Sleep
Sleep is increasingly recognized as a major factor in weight loss. We have a multitude of hormones that are affected by sleep, or lack thereof, and two of the most important are leptin and ghrelin. These two hormones are responsible for the feelings of satisfaction and fullness. If you do not get adequate sleep, whether alcohol was involved or not, you will eat more food the next day; this is a scientific fact. Quick tip: next time you have inadequate sleep, note

the difference in your appetite and the amount of food you consume or felt like consuming.

I hope this list achieved its goal, which is to give you a sense of being properly informed. It is pretty easy to see how alcohol can cause people to gain a lot of weight, and how regular consumption of alcohol would make losing weight very difficult. I'm a big believer in making decisions based on knowing the full picture and I think (actually I know) that many people are simply unaware of how damaging alcohol is to an effective weight loss plan. They may feel like they are doing everything they can by eating healthy and cutting sweets yet they are frustrated and eventually demotivated because they do not see results. The beauty of being knowledgeable on the subject is that you are fully aware of the trade-offs and implications. Knowledge truly is power - the power to make informed decisions about how you live your life.

A final few words on alcohol for women over the age of 40. Typically, less acidic drinks are better for you so I recommend red wine or vodka and club soda. Best to stay away from the sugary mixes and drinks made with milk and heavy creams, and remember that shots are generally very high in calories and therefore should be taken out of your diet permanently.

For men I have found that if you pay attention, even somewhat, to eating clean food and cutting out beer through the week you can have incredible weight loss. Since men have more muscle tissue than women they lose weight more easily because their body uses more energy, even at rest. Men can eat ten percent more than women and still lose weight faster, which isn't fair but it is what it is so let's just deal with it!

Alcohol can be a great part of our social lives. We just need to plan ahead for those events and drink in moderation.

CHAPTER SIX : Masterful Goal Setting

Goals are dreams with time frames matched to action.

Everyone has a vision for their health, wellness and fitness but some people never move past that dream state. If you are going to achieve the end result (which is your dream or your vision) you must progress to the next step by setting behavioural and cognitive goals. Effective goal setting has a number of key components and if any of these is missing you are less likely to manifest your overall vision for your health, wellness or fitness; this chapter will explore the components of masterful goal setting.

Step One: Readiness to change

All change has a predictable pattern; while you may be in the action stage in one area of your life (quitting smoking, for example), you may still be in the contemplation stage for another area such as losing weight. Here are the five stages of change:

1. Pre-contemplation

I can't/I won't. Where change can't even be considered because the person either doesn't want to, or believes for whatever reason that they cannot affect change in behaviour.

2. Contemplation

I may. Where there is consideration of what the change in behaviour may look like but there are no concrete plans just yet.

For people in the pre-contemplation and contemplation stage it is helpful to have cognitive, or learning, goals. The person in this stage of change may not be ready to act on a goal but they may find benefit and motivation by reading or gathering pertinent information.

3. Preparation

I will. Where preparation is underway, plans are being made and specific personal goals are being set.

4. Action

I am! Active participation in the process of change.

5. Maintenance

I still am. Where consistent maintenance of the new behaviour has been in place for at least 6 months.

It's important to identify where you are in your readiness to change a certain unhealthy behaviour, because your success ultimately depends on matching up your stage of change with the kinds of activities that will motivate you for the stage you are in. For example, you're a smoker and aren't even considering quitting but a loved one desperately wants you to stop. You're hounded and preached to about all the reasons you should quit but it doesn't motivate you; instead it turns you off and makes you angry. But let's consider for a moment that you're in the contemplation stage - you would be more ready to listen, and would be open to different choices. See the difference? You have to be ready for change in order for it to be successful.

Step Two: Write Down Your Vision

A vision is a detailed picture of your ideal self. How do you picture your life and who you want to be? What do you look like, and feel like? What are your dreams and heartfelt desires for your wellness, health and fitness? The vision needs to be as detailed as possible and spoken in the present tense, as if it's already who you are. You could create a vision using separate components or, as shown below, it can be a single all-encompassing vision complete with fitness, health and spiritual aspects. It's your vision of your ideal self as long as it reflects your heartfelt desires for you, anything goes.

I am at my healthy weight and size and I know this because I feel comfortable in my clothes and in expressing myself around friends and colleagues. My energy level is high and consistent throughout the day and I have plenty of energy for my work, children and spouse. I feel a sense of good health nearly all the time and I am free from aches, pains and sickness. I maintain above average health for my age. I feel content and fulfilled professionally and personally, and maintain feelings of peace and balance by doing yoga, lifting weights, doing cardio exercise and enjoying friends and the occasional glass of my favourite wine. I have a strong sense of purpose for my life and I continue to grow spiritually by reading my favourite authors and doing daily meditation.

Now this vision is the big picture. It may be a three-month plan or it may require a year or more to reach. Use the 0-10 scale to determine how large of a gap exists between where you are now and where you want to be; this will give you some measure of how long it will reasonably take to reach 70% or more of your ideal self as described in your vision.

When you are ready to set goals, use the SMART tool to ensure these goals are achievable.

S = specific. Include details such as when, where, how much, how long.
M = measurable. Make sure you can measure your goal; this is how you know you are being successful in reaching your goal.
A = action oriented. Your goals, whether they are thinking or doing goals, have to be action oriented.
R = realistic. The goal you choose must be realistic. If I had a goal of becoming an astronaut at the age of 49 that is probably not realistic, therefore I set myself up for failure not matter how hard I try.

T = timeline. Every goal must have a timeline associated with it otherwise there is no urgency.

An example of goal setting is as follows:

Goal/Desired outcome: lose 10 lbs

Action: Cardiovascular exercise 4 x per week for 1 hour duration. I will do moderate to high intensity and I will use a combination of the treadmill and outdoor walking

Action: I will eat clean food (no sugar or preservatives) 80% of the time, and will allow for either one special meal or one alcoholic drink each week (not both)

As you can see, the desired outcome is the goal but you need to go one step further and be specific with the action steps because a goal without action steps is almost certain to fail. How do you know when you're successful if you didn't put any measurable actions in place? This is a great example of why so many new year's resolutions do not come to fruition. They are usually stated as outcomes rather than actions.

Goals can also be cognitive or thinking goals. If, for example, you were not ready to begin action on a desired outcome or goal (managing stress effectively, for example) you could begin to gather information on managing stress instead, or read about ways to manage stress in a positive manner. Using the SMART goals tool, even for cognitive goals, increases the likelihood of success.

CHAPTER SEVEN : The Five Pillars of Successful Weight Loss

These pillars are the underpinnings of success as it relates to your weight loss and health goals. I can share all manner of tips, tricks and tactics but if you have not laid a rock-solid foundation from which to launch your weight loss plan, you simply will not have the success you are looking for. The clients who accept the pillars as the foundation on which all else is built have experienced magnificent transformations, because they understand that in order to do well, the foundation must be solid.

The pillars are used throughout the various stages of the weight loss process as well as for maintenance. For example, when you are writing your vision of your ideal self I want you to picture it with great detail. Your vision of your most ideal self should be so clear in your mind's eye that you can almost feel it; close your eyes and feel what it would be like and how your life would be better if you were to achieve this goal. When you are making your plan each week and organizing yourself for exercise and food preparation, you will have to prioritize your days and make critical decisions that allow you to meet your goals, and by adopting these pillars as your basic framework you will stay committed, organized and motivated. Clients often comment that even though they are not planners, the week moves ahead so much more easily when they have planned and prepared ahead. If something works and helps you achieve certain outcomes, use it!

Picture it
People who are mega successful and fulfilled have one thing in common: they have a vision! That vision is so clear and detailed it's like a GPS guiding them closer and closer to their goal. This is what you will need as you set your course on weight loss and a new body with improved health. You have to see it and feel it and know without a doubt that you can achieve it in order for it to manifest. No one else has to see your vision or believe in it but you must have a crystal clear vision of who you want to be, how you want to look, feel, act and be. We will further create this picture for you when we discuss creating your vision and setting goals, so you should start thinking about it now.

Prioritize
To reach your weight loss goals and maintain the weight loss forever you are most likely going to have to make some difficult choices about where you spend your time, and on what. You are going to have to clear the deck, as I like to call it, by assessing what is of utmost importance in your life and what can take a back seat, perhaps permanently. Think about what values you hold dear that need to be mirrored in your daily behaviours. For example, if you say you

want to lose 50 lbs but you continue to bring chips, pop and candy into the house instead of fruit and veggies you are not making your weight loss a priority. If you say that the health of your children is important to you yet they sit in front of the TV or computer for hours every day, you are not supporting that value of keeping your kids healthy. If you are going to lose weight it is going to take focus, planning, time and prioritizing. The only way you are going to be successful with your weight loss is if you accept the fact that everything associated with living a healthy lifestyle has to be top priority.

Planning and Preparation (success begins and ends here)
Few human endeavours are successful without a thorough plan, and weight loss is no exception. All my clients will tell you that the key to their successful weight loss is planning their meals and activities, then making the necessary preparations so they are not caught off guard. There's the expression "fail to plan, plan to fail" and this is absolutely on-point as it relates to losing weight. Unfortunately almost all overweight people hate to plan, and it's the reason why many of us stay that way. I will share fast and simple techniques that help you be prepared at all times.

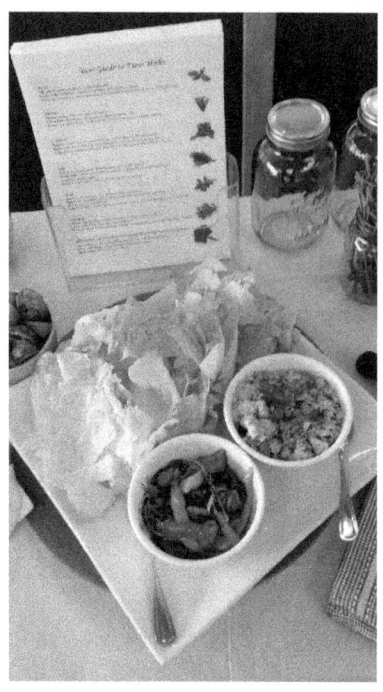

Ponder and Perfect

This is a very important step that barely exists in most, if not all, diet books. We live dynamic lives; our life situations change, jobs change, our children need change, the seasons change, nothing is static. What if you're humming along, losing weight, feeling great and possessing a strong sense of fulfillment about your achievements when life suddenly throws you a curve ball. Expected or not, you need to stop and reflect on what part of your plan is still working for you, as well as what needs adjustment, and then formulate a new plan. Simple. Be flexible and aware of changes in your day or your life so that you can accommodate them more easily with some brainstorming and creative tweaking.

PhD

To make weight loss a success over the long term, you need to stay interested and motivated in the kinds of things that help you to lose weight and live a healthy lifestyle, and the very best way to do this is to continuously find new things that you find intriguing and want to try. Remember, I am not selling a diet; instead, I'm introducing you to a way of thinking that is all about your behaviour. You are going to behave your way to being slim and healthy so you must find things that keep you wanting to pursue healthy eating and positive lifestyle choices, otherwise it is guaranteed you will go back to your earlier unhealthy habits.

Some of the ways I stay motivated some twenty years after losing weight include reading fitness and health magazines, attending lifestyle and health conferences, and surrounding myself with like-minded people who exercise and eat well. Annually, I create a vision board and keep it where I'm constantly reminded of my goals for myself. Perhaps you will follow in my footsteps and become a fitness instructor, or take a nutrition course so that you can help others. Whatever methods you use to stay tuned into your weight loss and healthy lifestyle is up to you; the important thing is to make sure you do something. Boredom and complacency will lead to relapse of unhealthy behaviour and weight gain.

CHAPTER EIGHT : 16 Power Habits

A habit is an acquired behaviour pattern regularly followed until it has become almost involuntary: the key word here is <u>regularly</u>. On the journey of weight loss and maintenance it's very important to lock onto the things that you know work in your favor and then do them every single day, no matter what. Throughout your weight loss you are going to find things that work well and help you to be successful. I encourage you to find your own habits but in the meantime I have formulated this list that clients and I have used with great success.

1. Get 6-8 hours of sleep each night. Sleep helps our body manage hormones that are associated with losing or gaining weight.

2. Drink 2-3 litres of water each day. Your body uses 2 Liters daily for bodily processes and if you exercise you require a bit more.

3. Keep your environment free of any trigger foods. You are less likely to eat something you don't want to if it's not in your house.

4. Eat a combination of protein and complex carbohydrates every 4 hours. Combining protein and carbohydrates helps keep you feeling full and energized.

5. Limit starchy carbohydrates to two half-cup servings per day. Foods like bread, rice, pasta, grains and potato are considered starchy because they quickly convert to sugar in the body, and what we don't use for energy is stored as fat.

6. Limit fruit to 2 servings per day. It's healthy but it's still sugar and we do not need much.

7. Incorporate exercise 4-6 times a week. Exercise is great for many health reasons but it's fantastic at helping you lose weight faster and keeping it off.

8. Journal all food: if you bite it, write it; if you nibble it, scribble it. If you are only eating fresh food in the proper portions you do not need to calculate calories but if you are eating out or eating a combination of packaged food and whole food then you may want to calculate your calories each day in your journal.

9. Eat healthy fats every day. Healthy fats such as nuts, avocados, peanut butter and seeds help satisfy your cravings and are essential for your brain, hair and skin.

10. Limit sugar from all sources to 25g per day. Basically your two servings of fruit is your sugar intake for the day. Beware of added sugar in packaged and processed food.

11. Plan ahead for meals and snacks. Do not wait until you are hungry to decide what your meal is going to be. That will cause you to make poor choices.

12. Carry food with you when you go out. Small food items like a banana or some almonds can help tide you over so that you are not starving.

13. Stand and move rather than sit. Being sedentary is very unhealthy. Be creative and find ways to stand and move rather than sitting still.

14. Add variety to your food and exercise to avoid boredom. Like many things in life you have to plan if you want to have fun. Plan your food and exercise a few days or a week in advance, and if something changes then work it into your plan.

15. Eat mindfully, and never in front of a TV, work station or other distraction. When you focus entirely on the food you are eating it gives your brain a chance to realize that you have eaten. You will eat less if you are mindful and present with your food.

16. Be accountable to a friend, group, or online program. It is necessary to have a support system to urge you on when you may not feel like continuing. If you know that someone else is counting on you then you are more likely to show up or do what you said you would do. I

have a workout buddy and we go to the gym at least 4 times each week together.

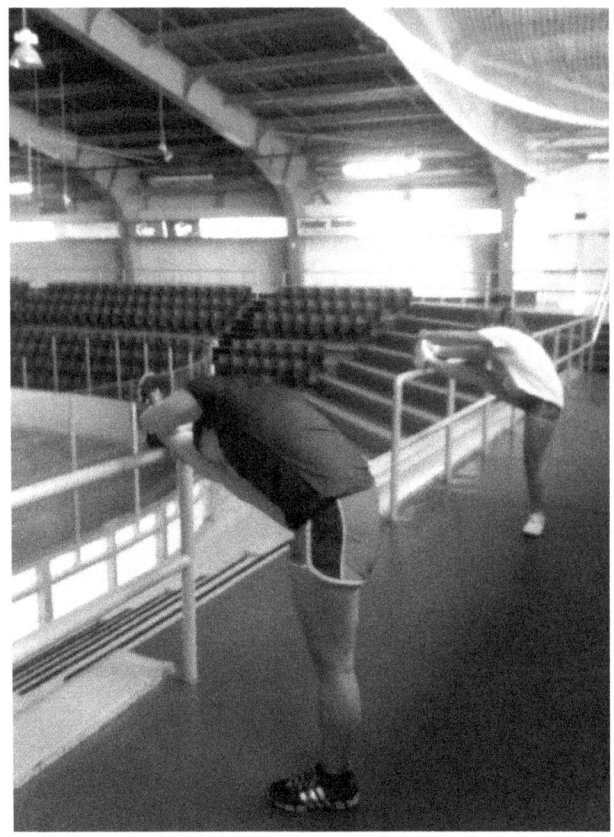

CHAPTER NINE : Plateau

Everyone who has ever started a plan to lose weight has come up against the dreaded plateau... that day when you step on the scale for your weekly weigh in and you didn't lose a single ounce. You beat yourself up because you did everything right, you exercised as usual and ate within your healthy calorie range and didn't cheat even once. You begin to have self-sabotaging thoughts and the downward spiral begins. The plateau, which can last days or weeks, can have a serious demotivating effect, causing you to eat badly and regain weight that you have worked so hard to lose.

I believe that knowledge is power and knowing why something is happening can provide a different perspective and serve to propel you forward. When you are initially losing weight you have a lot working in your favour: you have plenty of water held in your body tissue and so the first five or ten pounds may come off quite easy, and you have more total body mass so you burn more calories than if you weighed less. As you lose weight you have less water weight to lose and as your body gets lighter you are burning fewer calories overall.

The plateau is an exercise in patience. No pun intended! If you stay the course with healthy food choices and moderate exercise you will see the scale move in your favour. The plateau, or temporary delay, occurs because it's taking a bit longer for a pound of body fat to be lost. Remember that one pound equates to 3500 calories so for you to lose a pound of body weight you need to create a deficit of 3500 calories in your body. It would not be safe to achieve this by calorie restriction alone so a consistent combination of exercise and healthy diet is the solution. The worst thing you can do during a plateau is overeat. Don't let your mind play games with you; just continue to be consistent with a clean diet comprised mostly of fruits and vegetables, count your calorie intake and you will eventually see your weight loss resume. You have my word on that. Consistency is key.

The plateau is also a good time to revisit your attitudes and beliefs toward weight loss and health. If you are so consumed with the plateau and seeing the scale move downward that it prompts a junk food binge I would suggest that you think carefully about what you are really working towards. Do you plan to go back to your previous habits once the "diet" is over? Do you ever say to yourself "I can't wait until I reach my goal"? What do you think will change when you reach your goal? How prepared are you for the reality that you have to eat clean forever if you want the lost weight to stay lost? I would encourage you to look at the other reasons that you are eating healthy that may have nothing to do with weight loss, and stay focused on those during the plateau.

What other benefits are you realizing from a healthier diet? Do you have more energy to do the things you love? Do you simply feel healthier? Does your skin look more vibrant? Do you have fewer aches and pains? Do your kids, spouse or grandchildren notice that you are eating healthier food? This widening of your views on food and its benefits will help keep you on track and motivated in the absence of weight loss. Sure the weight loss is great; it's so rewarding to put in the effort with clean food and exercise and then see the number on the scale go down. However, it's also rewarding to feel better, feel healthier and set a positive example for the people in your life.

One last word on the weight loss plateau. I always ask my clients how they would gauge weight loss if scales did not exist. It may mean an increased sense of well-being, looser clothing, feeling good about the way you look, or smaller body measurements... there are so many other indicators that your body is changing for the better! Don't get hung up on the number on the scale as the only measurement of your success, remember to take into consideration all the other factors as well.

If you are doing resistance training as part of your weekly exercise routine then you are not going to see the scale drop as fast as someone who is not weight training. As you build muscle tissue you will look smaller because muscle takes up less room that fat, but muscle weighs more than fat so you look smaller but your actual weight may be a bit higher. Who cares! If you look amazing, feel awesome and have muscle tone it's all good.

CHAPTER TEN: Weekends, day trips & vacations

Most of us enjoy a little down time, some time away or just a small break from the monotony of the work week, because our vacations and weekends are a time to regroup and have fun. These changes to the normal routine can be stressful and even destructive if you have embarked on a weight loss journey.

When people begin a healthy diet and new exercise routine they frequently report that it is easy to follow their plan during the week but weekends, vacations and business travel wreak havoc with meals and food selection. The bad news is I personally experience the exact same challenges each time I travel or break my routine, but the really great news is that I have a plan for you.

The old saying 'fail to plan, plan to fail' couldn't be more true in this case. Just as you set goals and made initial plans to embark on your weight loss journey you must apply the same strategy to your weekends and travel time. The fact that you are at this point shows progress, right? If you are astute enough to recognize the problem before it's a problem then it's progress. It's progress if you have your healthy routine nailed down during the work week and now want to extend your healthy way of living to your leisure time.

On the flip side, if you are reading Curve Appeal from cover to cover and have not yet started your weight loss planning, it will be easy to incorporate the lessons from this chapter in your plans and goal setting. As you make plans to integrate healthy eating and exercise into your precious time I want you to remember this phrase: progress, not perfection.

It has been nearly 25 years since I lost weight and I am still finding new ways to better manage weekends and vacation time. You too will find things that work for you and things that don't; just keep what works and ditch what doesn't. My suggestions are just that, suggestions; you will come up with fun and creative ideas all your own... who knows, maybe I'll be reading your book someday!

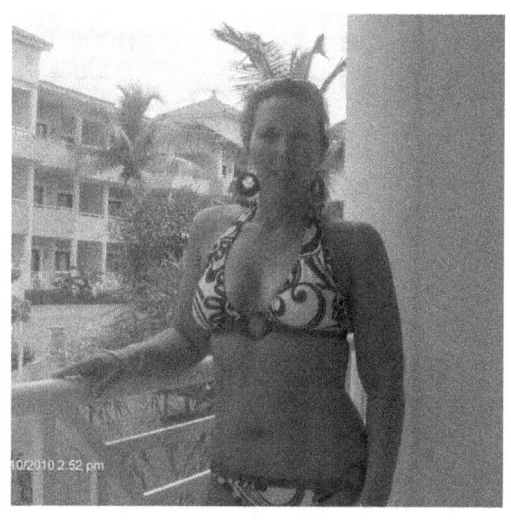

Vacations

If you have control of the vacation planning, you could consider a shift from the usual destinations and instead try an active and health-centered locale. Here are a few ideas:

Yoga retreat
Hiking and fishing lodge
Healing and natural medicine spa
Vacations that emphasize a healthy lifestyle such as tennis, horseback riding, snorkelling and other activities that keep you busy and away from the buffet table.

All-inclusive resorts and cruises can be a ton of fun but be very aware that there is food - free food - everywhere you turn. Free drinks too, depending on the package you purchased. Some survival tips:

Monitor your total daily calories and consume between 1200-1400

Buy a calorie counter book, or use an app, and take it everywhere

Choose food or alcohol but not both

Eat protein and fruit at breakfast because it will hold you over longer than carbohydrates such as toast and bagels (in my experience, resorts make amazing omelettes)

Eat fruits and salads during the day if you plan to eat a larger meal at supper

Exercise! This is the one instance where I suggest people over-exercise. Move, move, move! This will accommodate a little indulgence

Do not graze or snack

Choose lower calorie alcoholic drinks such as red wine, vodka and club soda or a light beer

Say no to all fruity cocktails. They are simple sugars

Drink three or more litres of water daily. You will sweat a lot so you need this much water to keep you hydrated and feeling full

Step out of your comfort zone and do things you typically would not do

Focus on friends, not food. Engage in conversation over a cold glass of sparkling water. It's just as much fun!

Tips for weekends & day trips

I had a client who had minimal success over the long term. She would lose 5 lb and then go away on a trip or a long weekend and put it back on; she'd reassure me that as soon as she was home and in a routine, she'd be fine. The problem was that she was never home for an extended stretch because her lifestyle consisted of constant travelling, so to be successful she would have had to find a way of eating clean and exercising while away. Hopefully some of my tips will make eating healthy on the road a bit easier.

Double up on a healthy protein-packed breakfast if you are running around all day with no plans to stop. One whole egg and a half cup of egg whites are great for an omelette

Always carry food in your purse or car such as nuts, bananas, apples, or homemade trail mix. Other options: Kashi brand bars, low fat cheese (1 oz or a cheese string), Greek yogurt, hard boiled egg

If you are unsure of dinner plans while away try eating mainly vegetables, salad and lean protein such as chicken or fish during the day to allow for a higher calorie meal at night

If you have more than one social event on a weekend you may have to choose just one to indulge in. Overeating and overdrinking at two events is enough to stall your weight loss for the upcoming week, and you may find you even gain a bit

Provide your own healthy foods if you are visiting someone's home

If dining out, ask the server to box up half of the carb portion before the meal is brought to the table

Call ahead to restaurants to inquire about low sodium and healthy options. Most of the time they are pleased to accommodate, especially with advanced notice

When stopping on the road for a meal, choose options that are known to you with ingredients that are familiar. Places like Subway offer a good selection and you are able to choose whether to hold the cheese, mayo and various toppings and condiments; load up on the lean protein and veggies instead, and say no to the meal deal

Decide ahead of time what you are committing to. If you wait until the trip is underway it's too late and you will make poor choices

Some people may suggest that you just relax, you're on vacation after all. Or you'll hear others saying how they simply wouldn't go on vacation if they couldn't eat and drink whatever they wanted. Don't let statements like these deter you or make you feel like you are taking your efforts too far; no one wants to return from vacation and face a weight gain of 5 lbs or more. Believe me, it's much easier to keep the weight off than it is to lose it time and time again. Remember that you are choosing to step away from the pack and to prevent the weight gain in the first place.

I want to encourage you to shift your perspective on this topic. Shift it from feeling sorry for yourself or feeling deprived, to feeling in control of the decisions that will support your weight loss and improved health. You are totally in the driver's seat and you are the only one who can get you where you want to go. When the trip is over, those around you will be impressed and wishing they had done the same thing.

With some attention to planning you will enjoy your weekends, vacations and a healthy happy weight.

NOW THAT'S HAVING IT ALL!

CHAPTER ELEVEN : Falling off the wagon

I would love to tell you that now that you are on your healthy eating plan and it's going well, you don't ever have to worry about lapsing or relapsing. I can't tell you that and it would be unprofessional of me to do so. Lapses are an expected part of any attempt at long term change. Change of any kind can be terribly difficult at times, and lapsing, albeit temporarily, is part of the process.

The reality of the situation is that someday, sometime you are going to momentarily ignore everything you have read in *Curve Appeal*, the advice and tips about planning and preparing and you are going to dive into your favourite food. It's that simple.

What isn't so simple are the numerous explanations of what brought you to that point. In this chapter I'm not going to get into all the possible ways to avoid this happening because no matter what we discuss as tools to avoid it, I can guarantee you 100% it is going to happen. Our time will be better spent discussing how to deal with these events in a way that strengthens you rather than leaves you for dead under the proverbial wagon to be run over again and again.

Even though I know exactly what makes me lapse from my own eating plan, it still happens from time to time. I know that when I am overtired, I cannot safely sit down to watch TV without snacking mindlessly. Once it happens I have two choices: 1) I can stop eating as soon as I become conscious of what I'm doing, go brush my teeth and fill my water bottle and get myself the heck out of the TV room. I can go log my extra calories and briefly write in my journal and move on. I can't change what I did but I can stop and regroup immediately. Not tomorrow, not next Monday or January 1st but right friggin now! or 2) I can, upon realizing what I'm doing, ignore it because I've already eaten half of the large bag of potato chips. I can beat myself up with terrible negative self-talk about what a loser I am and how once again I've let myself down. I can keep eating until the whole bag is gone and then convince myself that I've blown it, so even though this is Tuesday, I'll start again on Monday. By the time Monday rolls around I will have lapsed into old behaviours and most likely gained three or four pounds.

What I just described above is the all-or-nothing attitude and I see this every day in my coaching practice. People think in terms of all-or-nothing. I ate one chip, so I may as well eat chocolate for lunch and French fries and gravy for dinner. I want to encourage you to sharpen your awareness skill. I want you to become very aware of your actions and stop them at the first possible opportunity and then resume your healthier practices right then and there. You have not ruined everything, not even close if you get back on track right now. Not two days later or a week later or a month later.

This may help you a bit. There is a difference between a lapse and a relapse. A lapse is a small break from otherwise normal behaviour. Perhaps you're off plan for an hour or a day. It's normal for a lapse to occur once in a while. A relapse is a complete breakdown of the healthy behaviour for a period of months.

What you will find over time, if you are really paying attention, is that you get to know your own triggers better and better. You will begin to realize that there are certain people, situations or environments that, despite planning, will cause you to fall off the wagon. Learn what those emotional or environmental triggers are and although you can never completely eliminate an occasional lapse you can get far better at minimizing the damage.

It was when I was training for my first bodybuilding competition that I realized how much of a trigger that the TV was for me. If I'm overtired, there is something about watching TV that triggers an almost uncontrollable desire to nosh on food. Now that I know this, I can choose to get away from the TV and divert my attention to something else. Go fold laundry.

CHAPTER TWELVE : The rest is up to you.

As I write this chapter, I feel like a mother preparing to see her last child leave the nest. If you have raised children you know the feeling. You are confident that you've taught them plenty of life skills and you feel that you are a good influence on them and that they will be fine. Then in the very next breath you feel as if you could have done more, said more, or gave them even more tools to be successful. When push comes to shove and they finally do go out on their own, you are going to be delighted at how well they are applying all that they've learned to the real world. At the same time you will be happy to see that they still need you and come home looking for support and encouragement.

Your journey to weight loss and better health with this book is very much like that relationship that I just described. I could probably fill another book with more information about how to lose weight and keep it off successfully, and at the end of that book I would still be feeling the same as I do now. I have to trust that you've learned enough in this book to successfully get you to your weight loss goal and beyond. I also know that you will need and want to learn and grow beyond this book and that is a wonderful thing. When I began my own journey nearly 25 years ago I would never have dreamed that today I would still be learning and continuously changing my views on food, exercise and optimum health.

Unlike other "diet" books I may be the only author on the topic of weight loss that is not providing you, the reader, with a specific "diet" to follow. Now, before you throw the book down and demand a refund I promise to not leave you hanging. Trust me. Seriously though, this book is not about any particular diet but rather about consuming healthy foods in healthy portions in a consistent fashion. There is no end to this way of living therefore it's not a "diet". Unless you use the word "diet" to describe a healthy way of living. That is how I personally use the term "diet".

Typically when people go "on" a diet that indicates that at some point they will go "off" the diet and return to their unhealthy way of eating. This causes the weight regain and the cycle continues until the next sexy "diet" comes along. As you probably realize after reading this book, this is NOT my idea of a healthy way to achieve a desired body weight. You have, by now, begun to think about long-term behaviour change, and committing to doable goals and actions rather than following specific food regimen for 17 days, 30 days or something of that nature.

One of the reasons these diet books fail the reader over the long-term is because the reader is not learning strategies to change the underlying behaviours that cause them to overeat, eat mindlessly, eat too much, or eat to deal with stress or other emotions. So when the "diet" is done the dieter returns quickly to old behaviours that lead them back to old ways of eating.

Before you leave my nest and head out on your own I am going to provide you with step-by-step instructions to help you put all that you have read into practice. I am also going to provide you with general guidelines for food so that you feel confident about getting started with portions and total calorie intake.

Get Started NOW

- Create your vision – this is your mental picture of your ideal self. Who do you want to be? How do you want to look and feel? What do you value in your life that making changes to your weight and health will support? Be very specific.
- Set goals & actions – keep the outcome in mind and also be sure to describe what actions are going to get you to the outcome.
- Planning & preparation – Your goals, once developed, are going to require you to plan

carefully and make preparations to support your goals, such as time for exercise and food prep or meal planning, for example.

- Journal ALL of your food and activity.
- Paste a copy of your 16 power habits on the inside cover of your journal.

Food

The recommendations I'm about to share with you are ridiculously simple and will get you the lean and healthy body you have always wanted. That said, the world of food science changes on a daily basis and can be extremely complicated even for experts to stay on top of. There are so many choices that sometimes your confused mind does nothing because you don't know where to start.

In recent years, we have been told that we should follow a high-protein diet, low or no carbs, eat like cave men, stay away from sugar, go gluten free, too much fruit is bad and the list goes on and on. For each diet book there are as many suggestions as to what and how you should eat if you want to lose weight. From that regard my book is no different because I have my belief too about how to eat if you want to lose weight and achieve your healthy weight and size forever. My book is different though because my recommendations are not only for 17 days or a month but **forever**!

Let's dig in (pardon the pun).

- Plan all meals and snacks. Use magazines and online recipe sites for clean meals and snacks.
- Eat clean 90% of the time ie 6 days of the week eat food from natural sources (fruit, vegetables, meat, fish, poultry, nuts, seeds, beans, and healthy fats).
- 10% of the time enjoy a food that may come from restaurant or packaged foods.

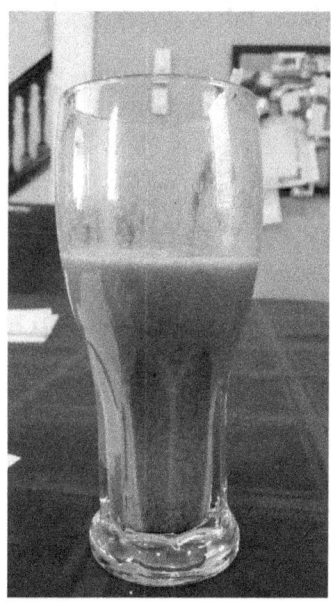

Follow these guidelines during your 6 days per week of clean eating:

1. Omit all *added* sugar.

2. Consume 10% of your total daily calories from healthy fat (natural peanut butter, olive oil, avocado, nuts and seeds). To calculate, take your total daily calories consumed multiplied by 0.10. If your daily calories for weight loss are 1300 then you should have 130 calories each day from healthy fats.

3. Eat plenty of vegetables - greens in particular.

4. Eat lean sources of protein such as chicken, lean beef or pork, salmon, haddock, cod, nuts, seeds, beans and plain Greek yogurt.

5. Drink 2-3 litres of water each day.

6. Omit drinks that contain artificial sweeteners.

You are on your way now.

I believe in you!

Other books published by Arcanum Acres Publishing:

The Natural Home Pharmacy

The Natural Home Pharmacy for Women

The Natural Home Pharmacy for Children

The Raw Milk Cleanse

The Path To Cure - The Whole Art of Healing Autism